What You Need To Know About Diabetes

What You Need To Know About Diabetes

OMIEPIRISA YVONNE BUOWARI

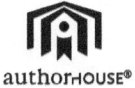

authorHOUSE®

AuthorHouse™ UK Ltd.
1663 Liberty Drive
Bloomington, IN 47403 USA
www.authorhouse.co.uk`
Phone: 0800.197.4150

Published by AuthorHouse   11/06/2013

ISBN: 978-1-4918-8289-4 (sc)
ISBN: 978-1-4918-8290-0 (e)

DEDICATION

This booklet is dedicated to diabetics and their care givers

PREFACE

Diabetes mellitus is a disorder caused by deficiency or diminished effectiveness of insulin in the body. It is associated with acute and long term problems involving the eyes, kidneys, nerves, blood vessels and other organs in the body. Insulin is a hormone produced by the pancreas that is important for regulating the amount of glucose in the blood. Glucose is a crucial source of fuel in the body and insulin facilitates the movement of glucose into cells. The red blood cells, healing wounds, brain and other organs in the body require glucose for fuel. Depending on the severity, diabetes mellitus is controlled with diet and exercise to lose weight, insulin or oral hypoglycaemic agents. Diabetes has some effects on the unborn baby during pregnancy therefore a pregnant woman who is diabetic is managed closely. Diabetes is a challenge during surgery as it requires close monitoring to ensure the blood glucose is within normal limits.

This book is to guide diabetics and help them to manage the disease effectively, control blood sugar, and prevent complications. This book should not be used as a substitute for diabetic therapy, self-diagnosis and medication. Diabetics should regularly visit their doctor and keep to advice and instructions.

Omiepirisa Yvonne Buowari

ACKNOWLEDGEMENTS

I wish to express my profound gratitude to all those who have contributed to making this work a success. I acknowledge all the agencies that provide free medical health care to rural Nigeria, through which I saw many undiagnosed diabetics. Some even have complications and they do not have access to health care because of poverty. Many diabetics do not have access to information on the disease. Some of these people have health care facilities around them but refuse to utilise them because of poverty and faith in traditional medicine.

I want to thank all those I came across who inspired me in the course of this work. This book would not have been a reality without the invaluable contributions of some special people who criticized and made useful recommendations, which have been considered and incorporated in the final script. Dr Datonye D. Alasia, Dr Tamunokuro Ezekiel Diamond, Dr Ikechi Amadi, and Dr Hilary Edgcombe are highly appreciated for proof reading the manuscript. Dr Nimi Stephanie Ekere is acknowledged for her passion in caring and educating diabetics. This book is a result of that vision when I planned to write a flier on diabetes mellitus for her. I thank all my teachers at my different levels of education, who have groomed me to what I am today. I wish to thank all the doctors I have worked with during my internship who taught me how to practice and implement all I learnt in the medical school on the management of the diabetic.

My special thanks also go to Dr Humphrey Igwacho and Dr Hope I Bellgam. I will not forget the families of Andrew Furo Green and Abel Thomas Jumbo of Grand Bonny Kingdom into which I was born for being there for me always and moulding me from cradle to adulthood.

I thank Dr Jachin Velavan of the Christian Medical College, Vellore, India for writing the foreword. Dr Jachin Velavan is involved in training general practitioners in distance fellowship diabetes management through distance education program and has evolved 10 self-learning modules. Last of all, I thank the Almighty God for helping me to complete this book and using me as an instrument in this regard.

FOREWORD

The International Diabetes Federation in its position statement on Diabetes mellitus talks about Diabetes self-management education (DSME) as a 'right for all'. Disseminating the right information and increasing awareness about diabetes definitely seem to be the way forward. With Diabetes reaching pandemic proportions, with a current global prevalence of about 170 million and an expected rise to about 370 million by the year 2030, there needs to be a sense of urgency in which information is shared both far and near, in big and small ways. I am delighted that Dr. Buowari has responded to this need and has compiled this book on diabetes to equip diabetics and their carers in what they need to know about diabetes which will undoubtedly help in more effective self-management of diabetes. It is an easy-read and I am sure will be useful to the target group.

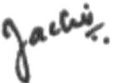

Dr. Jachin Velavan
MBBS, DNB (Fam Med), M.R.C.GP. (Int)
Family Physician & Coordinator
Department of Distance Education
Christian Medical College
Vellore, Tamilnadu, India.
September, 2012.

CONTENTS

CHAPTER 1

WHAT IS DIABETES?

There are two types of diabetes, namely diabetes mellitus and diabetes incipidus. Diabetes insipidus is a disorder in which there is production of large quantities of dilute urine and constant thirst due to the deficiency of a hormone (chemical) known as vasopressin (also known as antidiuretic hormone) produced by the pituitary gland. Glands are organs in the body that produce chemicals known as hormones in the body. A hormone is a substance that is produced in one part of the body, passes into the bloodstream and is carried to other organs or tissues where it acts to modify their structure or function. Vasopressin regulates the reabsorption of water in the kidneys. The focus of this book is Diabetes mellitus.

Definition of Diabetes Mellitus

It is a disorder in the breakdown of food compounds in which sugars in the body are not processed to produce energy due to lack of insulin. The accumulation of sugar in the body leads to its appearance in the blood (hyperglycaemia), then in the urine. The symptoms of diabetes mellitus include thirst, loss of weight and the excessive production of urine.

Insulin and What It Does

Insulin is a hormone (chemical) produced by an organ in the body called the pancreas that is important for regulating the amount of sugar (glucose) in the blood. The pancreas lies just behind the stomach. Insulin is released into the blood stream to escort glucose from the blood to the cells. When it is working correctly, the sugar that comes into the blood stream can go right into the cells of the body. Insulin helps the glucose to enter the cells where it is used as fuel by the body. It promotes carbohydrate utilisation and regulates energy production, storage and release. All actions of insulin are concerned with storage and breakdown of absorbed nutrients. A diabetic either produces virtually no insulin, or produces what does not function properly, or produces insulin that cannot be utilized by the tissues. Where insulin is produced by the body and it cannot be utilized by the tissues of the body, it is known as insulin resistance. The body produces more insulin after a meal to reduce the amount of glucose in the food ingested.

Causes of Diabetes Mellitus

The cause may be unknown but it may be inherited or due to disease of the pancreas and drugs. It may be due to other conditions. Diabetes occurs either because of lack of insulin or because of the presence of factors that oppose the action of insulin.

Importance of Glucose in the Body

Glucose is the final product of all carbohydrate that is eaten such as rice, potatoes, sugar, and other sweet foods which contain pure sugars like ice cream. Glucose is an important source of energy. The tissues of the brain, kidney and the red blood cells depend entirely on glucose as a source of energy. Therefore, the control and balance of glucose levels in the body is important to life. Carbohydrates are abundant in most meals. Carbohydrates play important roles in the nutrition of man. They are important in the diet and supply much of the energy needed commonly referred to as calories. Starch is the major carbohydrate component of many foods, such as rice, bread, corn etc. Once a meal is eaten, the glucose produced by digestion of the food is absorbed into the blood stream and its concentration increases. The World Health Organisation Expert Committee on Diabetes Mellitus describes the disease in terms of blood glucose level.

Types of Diabetes Mellitus

There are two main classes of diabetes mellitus, namely:

- **Type I Diabetes Mellitus also known as Insulin Dependent Diabetes Mellitus (IDDM):** It is due to the deficiency of insulin. Diabetics with this type require administration of insulin.
- **Type II Diabetes Mellitus also known as Non-Insulin Dependent Diabetes Mellitus (NIDDM):** It is due to reduced production of insulin or resistance to insulin. These diabetics are placed on drugs known as oral hypoglycaemic agents that potentiate the action of insulin.

Diabetes mellitus is an incurable disease but it can be controlled and affects both adults and children. Without treatment after a meal, the amount of glucose in the blood would rise that could eventually damage the heart, kidneys, eyes, and nerves. People who do not have diabetes have a constant level of insulin produced. The sufferer manages the disease throughout his/her lifetime. Diabetes may be controlled on diet alone. It may also require administration of drugs that is tablets and insulin injection to maintain satisfactory control.

Symptoms of Diabetes Mellitus

- Excessive urination.
- Excessive thirst due to loss of fluid.

- Weight loss while eating good food from breakdown of tissue due to less glucose in the cells and hence increased utilisation of protein for energy. Weight loss due to other conditions such as malnutrition should also be considered.
- Excessive eating.

The above are the major symptoms. There are other minor ones as well which include the following:

- Ants gathering on urine
- Tiredness
- Blurred vision
- Frequent skin, bladder and gum infection
- Irritability
- Tingling sensation in the hands and feet
- Slow and poor healing of wounds
- Sometimes may involve the food passage leading to diarrhoea
- Genital itching

During fasting, glycogen stored in the liver is transformed into glucose but it is rapidly depleted within hours. Insulin secretion is reduced. Therefore, if a diabetic must fast, it should be under the guidance of a doctor because starvation in the diabetic can give rise to high levels of sugar in the blood.

CHAPTER 2

MANAGEMENT OF DIABETES MELLITUS

Diabetes mellitus is diagnosed from the individual's complaints and tests carried out. The test done to diagnose diabetes mellitus are random blood sugar, fasting blood sugar, two hours post prandial, oral glucose tolerance test and urine test. Other tests are done to support those mentioned above. When high blood sugar is noticed from routine test carried out without symptoms, a confirmatory test is done.

Laboratory Tests

- **Fasting blood sugar**: The individual fasts overnight and the blood sugar is tested in the morning before taking a meal.
- **Random blood sugar**: The blood sugar is tested at any time of the day.
- **Two hours post prandial**: The blood sugar is tested two hours after eating.
- **Oral glucose tolerance test**: An overnight fast is done for at least ten hours but not more than sixteen hours. Water but no beverage is allowed. Blood sample is withdrawn and the blood glucose estimated. A solution of 75g of glucose in 300mls of water is drunk. Blood samples for blood sugar estimation are collected at 30 minutes, 60minutes, 90 minutes and 120 minutes after drinking the glucose solution.
- **Glycosylated haemoglobin**: This is a stable form of the haemoglobin which is present in the blood in proportion to the

average blood glucose level overtime. Haemoglobin is a substance contained within the red blood cells responsible for their colour. It has the unique property of combining reversibly with oxygen and is the medium by which oxygen is transported within the body. This is the best marker for recent blood glucose control.

The glucometer is a simple handy machine useful and sensitive for the measurement of blood sugar levels. It can be used for home monitoring of diabetes. It has strips and lancing devices for piercing the skin.

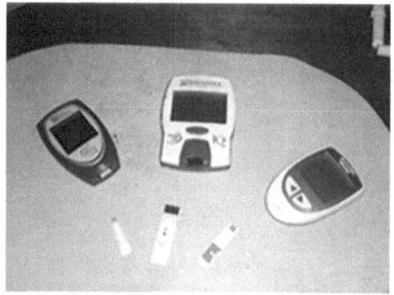   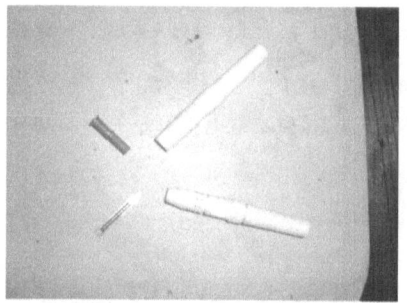

Different brands of glucometers   Lancing devices and lancets

Treatment

Most times people are shocked when told they are diabetic. There is no cure for diabetes mellitus but it can be controlled so that the individual can enjoy a healthy life. This is to help keep the blood sugar level near to normal. Together with a healthy lifestyle, this helps to improve the well-being of the person and protect against long-term damage to the eyes, kidneys, nerves, hearts and blood passages. The diabetic plays an important role in the care and treatment of the disease.

The aims of treatment are to:

- To save life
- To abolish symptoms
- To prevent long term complications and treat if present
- To educate diabetics about the disease
- Encourage self management
- To attain and maintain optimal bodyweight
- To provide a state of wellbeing
- To provide emotional support
- To achieve a normal physical and emotional growth in diabetic children
- To keep the kidneys functioning well
- To control blood pressure if the diabetic is also hypertensive
- To prepare for pregnancy and have good outcome
- To provide optimal nutrition

The diabetic team comprises of the following:

- Physician
- Dietician
- Podiatrist (doctor that cares for the feet and treat foot diseases)
- Diabetic educator
- Social worker
- Ophthalmologist
- Pharmacist
- Obstetrician (for pregnant women)

Podiatry is the branch of medicine devoted to the study, diagnosis and treatment of disorders of the foot, ankle and lower leg. The physician aims at providing a comprehensive care for diabetics and devices a management plan on the blood sugar control. The diabetes educator is a health worker who teaches people with diabetes how to manage the disease.

The components of diabetic treatment are:

- Education
- Counselling
- Monitoring
- Drugs
- Dietary control

Dietary control and regular exercise is important in diabetic control. Diabetic diet is the best diet for the general population. All diabetics need careful continuous dietary regulation and adjustment. Dietary management is essential in the treatment of diabetes. A diabetic cannot balance the sugar in the blood quickly but still needs energy. Choose food that is high in fibre as these allow sugar to be absorbed more slowly. This alone may be adequate to achieve and maintain normal blood glucose levels. Meals should be balanced, contain high fibre diet and low in fat. Alcoholic drinks are high in calories; do not substitute them for meals. Eat less fried and fatty foods. Sugars have to be taken away from the diet. The amount of starchy food eaten should be reduced but not totally removed from the diet. Protein should be taken as required for the age. The diabetic have to give up smoking and drinking alcohol.

Avoid
- ☒ Any form of sugar
- ☒ Drinks containing sugar
- ☒ Glucose
- ☒ Sweet biscuit
- ☒ Chocolates

☒ Cakes
☒ Beverages
☒ Ice cream

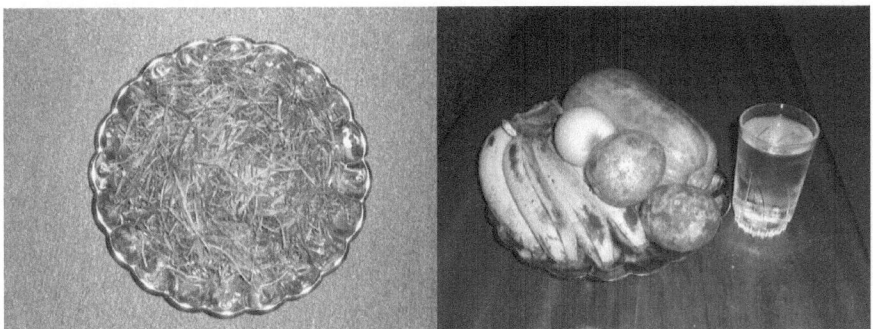

Fruits and vegetables taken as desired

Physical activity is an important part of managing diabetes. It helps to regulate blood sugar levels, helps insulin to work effectively and reduces the risk of heart disease, high blood pressure, and stroke. The blood sugar levels can be kept within recommended limits by combining diabetes treatment with healthy diet, regular physical activity, and weight control.

When an individual is managed on diet alone without control, drugs are introduced depending on the blood sugar level. The doctor decides on which is suitable for a particular individual. These drugs have toxic and fatal side effects if taken by non-diabetics. A medical practitioner should always prescribe them. It should not be bought over the counter without a doctor's prescription, or when noticing symptoms same as someone that has been diagnosed diabetic by a medical doctor.

These tablets are known as oral hypoglycaemic agents. They should be taken with meals. When missed for any reason, it should not be taken with the next dose. Pregnant women should not take the tablets because they can cause congenital malformation in the baby.

In pregnancy, these oral hypoglycaemic drugs are stopped and insulin injection administered till delivery. Some of the side effects of these oral hypoglycaemic agents are:

- Low blood sugar that persist for many hours and should be treated in hospital
- Weight gain
- Can lead to kidney problem
- Vomiting and feeling like vomiting(nausea)
- Facial flushing after drinking alcohol
- Skin reaction
- Fever
- Affects the liver leading to liver failure
- Occasional interaction with drugs taken for other conditions

Another drug for the treatment of diabetes mellitus is insulin. This is an injection given under the skin. The individual is taught how to inject him or herself. Insulin is taken thirty minutes before food. The food must be ready before taking the drug. If taken without food, the blood sugar drops and the individual collapses. The following groups of diabetics are likely to need insulin injection:

- Children
- Pregnant women
- Diabetics whose treatment with tablets have failed
- Individuals who for any reasons have their pancreas removed (pancreatectomy)
- Diabetic foot ulcer

There are three main types of insulin delivery systems:

- Vial and syringe
- Insulin pen which may be reusable injection pen or disposable pen
- Insulin pump

The best place to inject insulin is in the fatty areas of the abdomen, buttocks and thigh. Do not inject in the same spot all the time as it can cause lumps in the skin. These lumps stop the insulin from working properly. Insulin is stored in a refrigerator. When purchasing insulin, always note the expiry date and name of insulin on its package. Reusable pen devices, needle and syringes should be stored carefully. Insulin is a hormone and should always be kept in a refrigerator. Needles should be disposed carefully. When travelling, insulin should be kept in a cooler or vacuum flask to preserve its potency.

Do not:

- Freeze insulin
- Keep insulin under direct sunlight
- Keep insulin in a hot place
- Use insulin that is lumpy or has changed colour
- Use insulin after the expiry date

When ill:

- Never stop taking drugs
- Test the blood glucose more frequently
- Rest
- Eat regular meals

➢ Consult a doctor if:
- Diarrhoea occurs
- Cannot eat for 24 hours
- High temperature(fever) occurs
- Blood glucose level continues to be high

The co-operation of the diabetic is highly essential for the management of the disease. Home monitoring should be done.

Home Monitoring

Testing of urine and blood sugar regularly at home is important. Urine testing can be done with reagent strips, which detect all reducing sugars. This does not give a true value of what is happening in the blood. Some other urine strips also test for leucocytes, urobilinogen, bilirubin, blood, nitrite, pH, specific gravity, protein, and ketones. The individual immerses the reagent strip into urine for approximately five seconds or as specified by the manufacturer. The colour of the reagent areas of the strip is compared with the colour chart on the label of the reagent strip container.

Diabetics can monitor their blood sugar at home. Blood sugar level gives a direct measure of the sugar level at the time and can detect low blood sugar. Blood sugar monitoring is best carried out by means of a meter called glucometer. It can be carried around. The blood sugar level will tell the effect of the treatment. Always go with a logbook used for recording the home blood sugar levels when going to see a doctor.

The purposes of home blood sugar measurement are:

- To measure changes of blood sugar
- To assess blood sugar control in times of special need

- To detect low(hypoglycaemia) and high (hyperglycaemia) blood sugar levels
- To obtain a full blood sugar profile
- Testing can be done at different times of the day. It is also necessary when there is a change in the normal routine, like before and after sporting activities, when travelling, and before and after special occasions like parties.

To perform home monitoring of the blood sugar, get the necessary materials like the glucometer, lancet, and test strip.

- Wash your hands. If cold, wash in warm water
- The glucometer should be on with the strip inside the machine before pricking to drop blood on the strip
- Put on the glucometer and follow the directions of the manufacturer
- When using a lancet, prick the side of the finger
- Record the result
- Dispose off the lancet safely

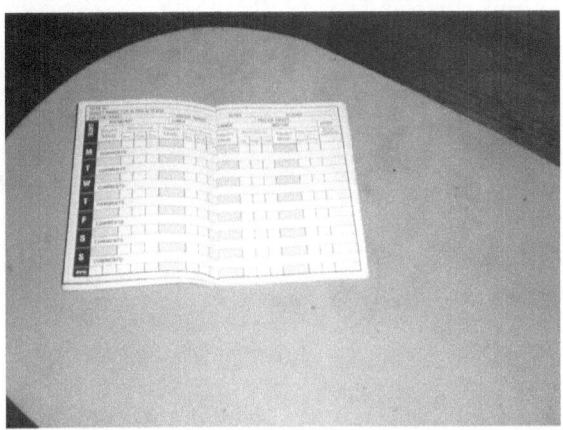

Log book for recording blood glucose values

There are different brands of glucometers and they are easy to operate. Some give an alarming warning sign when the blood sugar is too high or too low, such as "Call Doctor Urgently", showing on the screen.

Foot Care

Diabetics need special care of their feet to avoid developing diabetic foot. Diabetic foot ulcer when discovered early and treated aggressively may heal without undergoing amputation.

- Daily foot checks
- Daily washing of the feet
- Check for signs of infection
- Do not use sharp instruments on the feet, avoid direct heat and hot water because of loss of pain and temperature sensitivity
- Wear well fitting shoes. Avoid tight shoes
- Avoid going around barefooted
- Check inside shoes and socks for sharp objects
- Avoid foot injury
- Report foot changes early to the doctor

CHAPTER 3

COMPLICATIONS OF DIABETES MELLITUS

Complications are worsening states that can follow the presence of a disease. Complications of diabetes mellitus can occur often when the diabetes is not under control. Sometimes the complication makes the person visit the hospital before a diagnosis of diabetes mellitus is made. Complications can arise from the disease itself or following treatment.

There is increased risk of disease of the heart and blood vessels (cardiovascular disease). Diabetics with long standing disease may develop complications affecting the eyes, kidneys, nerves, or major arteries. Detection of early signs of complications of diabetes mellitus is an essential requirement of diabetes care, leading to early prevention and treatment strategies, which can abort progression of some of the most serious consequences. One of the most dangerous and dreaded complication of diabetes is diabetic coma.

Diabetic Ketoacidosis

This is the most common complication of diabetes mellitus and is shortened as DKA. Carbohydrate is necessary for the complete breakdown of fats in the body. When there is a disorder in the breakdown of carbohydrate, the breakdown of fat is incomplete and intermediate products (ketones) can accumulate in the blood leading to what is known as ketosis. These ketones make their breath to be sweet smelling. The breakdown of protein in this situation leads to weight loss, and contributes to the development of weakness and high blood sugar levels. Ketones are very harmful and the body will immediately try to get rid of them by excreting them in urine. The ketones can be detected by the use of a type of strip used in testing urine samples. Ketones are not present in the urine of normal healthy individuals. They are present in the urine of uncontrolled diabetes, prolonged fasting or persons consuming high fat and low carbohydrate diet. Diabetic ketoacidosis can occur in both adults and children. It is a serious illness, which requires hospital admission. It is precipitated by:

- Infections of any kind
- Trauma
- Surgery
- Uncontrolled diabetes
- Interruption of insulin therapy
- Stress of inter-current illness

The symptoms of diabetic ketoacidosis are:

- Excessive urination, thirst and hunger
- May present for the first time
- May have obvious evidence of infection or trauma
- May be complaining of abdominal pain
- Vomiting
- Extreme weakness
- Drowsiness and dizziness
- Unconsciousness
- Skin, tongue and mouth may be dry
- The eyes may sink inside
- The breath may have a fruity smell
- Deep rapid breathing.

Diabetic ketoacidosis is an emergency and should not be managed at home. The person should be taken immediately to the hospital. The blood sugar level is restored back to normal by administration of insulin. Any infection is treated with antibiotics. Death can result if left untreated.

Hyperosmolar Hyperglycaemic State/Non-Ketotic Hyperosmolar Coma:

It has a slow progression with the person finally loosing consciousness. It is a less common condition and is precipitated by:

- Infections
- Other inter-current diseases
- Consumption of foods rich in glucose

Lactic Acidosis

This may occur due to shock, exercise, drugs, chemicals, toxic compounds, severe liver disease etc.

Diabetic ketoacidosis, hyperosmolar hyperglycaemic state, lactic acidosis and low blood sugar (hypoglycaemia) can cause unconsciousness (coma).

Complications Affecting the Blood Passage

Diabetes can affect the blood vessels giving rise to stroke.

Eye Problems

This may be due to cataracts or retinopathy that damages the back of the eye. They lead to visual changes and diminishing vision. There are changes in the sizes of objects and difficulty in the differentiation of colours. This may lead to blindness. Diabetes can also cause cataract. This can be prevented by control of diabetes and regular eyes checks and screening. Treatment prevents the eyesight from becoming worse, but may not restore vision already lost.

Nephropathy

This is damage to the kidneys. Kidney damage is made worse by high blood pressure. Diabetes mellitus can make the kidneys to stop working properly. If untreated, it leads to kidney failure, a condition where the kidney cannot function properly.

Infections

- Skin infections giving rise to boils and abscesses
- Infections of the mouth
- Periodontal disease leading to loss of teeth
- Uncontrolled diabetes can cause tooth decay
- High blood sugar damages the blood vessels in the mouth. This will reduce the flow of oxygen and nutrients to the gum, thereby weakening their ability to fight against infection.

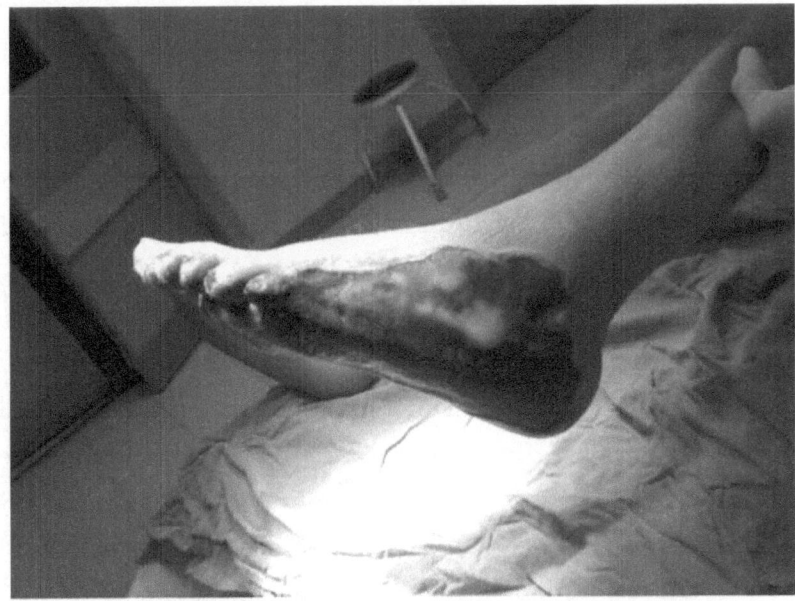

Leg ulcer following uncontrolled diabetes mellitus

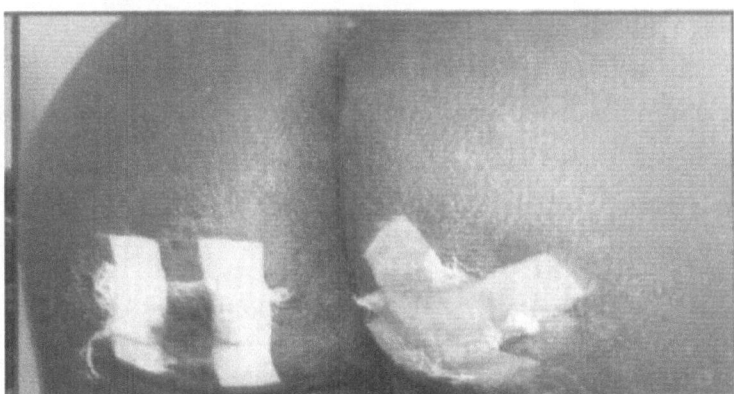

Chronic ulcers (wound) on the buttocks following uncontrolled diabetes

Neuropathy

Neuropathy is any disease that affects the peripheral nerves and it can be caused by diabetes. Pain is the chief symptom. Cramping pain and weakness of the muscles occur. Neuropathy means damage to the nerves of the body.

Nerves are thread-like structures which carry hundreds of thousands of tiny fibres, linking all parts of the body inside and outside to the brain. They carry tiny signals of information back and forth, making it possible for us to feel and move. The brain is the central control room of all our bodily actions and sensations. Information back and forth in the brain passes up and down the spinal cord and out through the peripheral nerves in the arms and legs for movements, actions, sensations and pain.

There are sensory and autonomic neuropathies. Sensory neuropathy is the most common type and the feet are most likely to be affected. There is loss of feeling in the feet. Autonomic neuropathy is less common. It affects the organs, which work without us being aware, such as the stomach, heart, bladder, sexual organs etc. Delayed emptying of the stomach can occur if there is damage to the nerves of the stomach resulting in early satiety, vomiting, nausea, discomfort and weight loss.

Diabetic Foot Ulcer

It is an ulcer in diabetics from infection, trauma, or pressure. The ulcer/wound is on the foot especially the first big toe. It is deep and punched out. Infection may spread and even precipitate loss of blood supply to the foot giving rise to what is known as gangrene. Gangrene is the death or decay of part of the body due to deficiency or cessation of its blood supply. This diabetic gangrene tends to start from one foot, usually after a minor injury. If this injury is left untreated, it can lead to loss of that foot or entire limb. Once this is noticed, the individual should report to the hospital where it will be examined by a medical doctor and the best decision concerning the situation will be taken. Insulin is administered. If the individual is on tablets (oral hypoglycaemic drugs), it is converted to insulin until the wound heals. Antibiotics are given to combat any infection and dressing of the wound is done daily.

If the blood supply is adequate then the dead tissues can be removed in the expectation that healing will occur provided infection is controlled and the foot is protected from pressure. Amputation is done if gangrene has occurred. This is difficult to accept. In some cultures, amputees are not given befitting and decent burials. In some others, amputees are not buried in their hometown, hence refusal to give consent for amputation in such societies and communities. Artificial limbs (prosthesis) and rehabilitation are expensive and not readily available in some countries. However people should be encouraged to have them, as it will help them return to their normal way of life before the amputation and improve the quality of life of the amputee.

Amputation sometimes can be preventable. Good care saves the leg. Amputation negatively imparts on the self-image and mobility of the individual. The surgery sometimes is done to preserve life and remove threatening limbs. It is accepted most times on the grounds of life threatening toxicity or unbearable offensive odours.

The care of the foot is very important and any wound must be treated aggressively. Amputation affects the quality of life.

Complications from the Treatment of Diabetes Mellitus

These complications arise from the treatment of diabetes.

Hypoglycaemia (low blood glucose): Hypoglycaemia is low levels or deficiency of sugar (glucose) in the bloodstream, causing muscular weakness and incoordination, mental confusion and sweating. It is treated by the administration of sugar (glucose). Low blood sugar levels results from:

- Overdose of insulin or tablets used in the treatment of diabetes
- Injection of insulin without food
- Sometimes it is caused by strenuous exercise
- Alcohol, stress or illness

Symptoms of Low Blood Sugar (Hypoglycaemia)

- Feeling of emptiness
- Weakness
- Hunger
- Nervousness
- Sweating
- Feeling of the heart beat(palpitation)
- Cold
- Dizziness
- Tiredness
- Confusion
- Fainting attack
- Headache
- Visual disturbances
- Loss of consciousness (coma)

- Double vision
- Incomprehensible speech

If low blood sugar (hypoglycaemia) is untreated, it can lead to permanent brain damage. It is more dangerous than high blood sugar. It can occur several hours after vigorous or prolonged exercise due to continuing uptake of glucose by the muscles. In children, vomiting, jerking of the limbs and convulsion can occur. Treatment is by consumption of simple sugar. If unconscious, the diabetic should be rushed to the hospital. The diabetic should consume sugar or glucose once consciousness is regained. Eat or drink something containing sugar immediately.

Skin Complications

- Painful lumps at the site of repeated insulin injections
- Loss of the fat under the skin at insulin injection sites leading to what is known as lipodystrophy
- Allergy at injection site

Other Complications

- Insulin resistance
- Weight gain

CHAPTER 4

DIABETES AND PREGNANCY

Diabetes mellitus is the most common medical complication of pregnancy, and it carries a significant risk. During pregnancy, the baby obtains glucose from its mother through the placenta. Sugar (glucose) in urine during pregnancy is not diagnostic of diabetes mellitus, nor can it be used as a monitor of diabetes. Two episodes however are regarded as an indication for blood sugar (glucose) test.

The progressive increase in insulin demand during pregnancy can make latent diabetes appear. This may resolve after the pregnancy. Some women show a slightly impaired glucose tolerance during pregnancy with reduction to normal condition after delivery.

Certain women are at special risk of developing diabetes during pregnancy. They are those who have:

- diabetes in a first degree relative
- recurrent miscarriages
- unexplained stillbirth
- previous baby with congenital abnormality
- previous very large baby
- previous diabetes in pregnancy
- persistent glucose in urine
- obesity.

All women who have had gestational diabetes mellitus, particularly those who are overweight are encouraged to keep to their diet for the rest of their lives regardless of whether their glucose tolerance test is normal or not. In the early stages of pregnancy, diabetic control may be complicated by nausea and vomiting. The mother needs more carbohydrate as the baby is growing. Ketosis is induced more easily particularly in the later stages of pregnancy. The diabetic who is being controlled by diet alone may become dependent on insulin. Women who have had diabetes since childhood and already have nephropathy and retinopathy must be monitored carefully for signs of deterioration. There are three classes of diabetes mellitus in pregnancy:

Established Diabetes: These women have been diagnosed to be diabetic before pregnancy. She is already aware of her condition and on diabetic drugs.

Gestational Diabetes: These women are healthy before pregnancy. They are diagnosed as diabetic during pregnancy. After delivery, the woman returns to her normal state. Some of these women later on in life may develop diabetes. Gestational diabetes may develop about midway through a pregnancy. It is caused by changes in the body messenger chemicals during pregnancy. The placenta also produces hormones. Women with gestational diabetes tend to have recurrent diabetes during subsequent pregnancies. Many women have no symptoms. The woman has to be followed up after delivery.

Impaired Glucose Tolerance: This woman shows an impaired glucose tolerance test. They are not diagnosed to be diabetic.

During pregnancy, there is relative insulin resistance by producing more insulin and releasing it at increased rates. Persistent high blood sugar (glucose) level in the mother causes high blood sugar level in the baby because glucose crosses from the mother's blood through the placenta to the baby, but insulin does not cross the placenta from the mother's blood to the baby's blood.

During Pregnancy:

- Diabetes tend to worsen
- Blood sugar control becomes difficult
- High blood sugar becomes frequent
- Organ damage becomes more common
- High risk of having infections such as infection of the urinary passage
- High blood pressure in pregnancy tends to occur
- The placenta is unusually large

The Antenatal Period

The woman is seen frequently than other clients. She may be admitted at any time she has an infection or the blood sugar control becomes difficult. She does a blood sugar (glucose) test any time she goes to the clinic. Women who are newly diagnosed may sometimes be admitted to bring down the blood sugar.

Effect of Diabetes on Pregnancy

- High rate of loss of pregnancy
- Big baby which may lead to difficult labour
- Delayed maturity of the baby's lungs
- Increased risk of pre-eclampsia secondary to increased placenta bulk

- Too much water for the baby in the womb
- Infections

The effects of diabetes mellitus on pregnancy may be minimal if the diabetes is well controlled. If the control is inadequate, there may be complications. The haemoglobin of the mother can become irreversibly bound to glucose. This is termed glycosylated haemoglobin.

The Effect of Pregnancy on Diabetes

The main effect is increased resistance to insulin. This makes the woman to require more insulin than she normally does. This requirement will return to normal once the woman is delivered of her baby. There is the risk of having the baby before the expected date of delivery because of too much water in the womb (polyhydramnios).

Effect of Diabetes on the Baby

Babies of mothers with poorly controlled diabetes may be large. The baby responds to the extra sugar by producing more insulin, which can increase its body fat and muscle mass. The head circumference and brain size are normal. After birth, the baby continues to produce more insulin than needed. Since there is no more supply of high levels of sugar from the mother, low blood sugar (hypoglycaemia) levels may occur. The baby's blood sugar level should be monitored after delivery. If the baby's blood sugar is unstable, the baby may be admitted to the hospital nursery (special care baby unit) for monitoring. All the serious effects of diabetes may be reduced by having good blood sugar control.

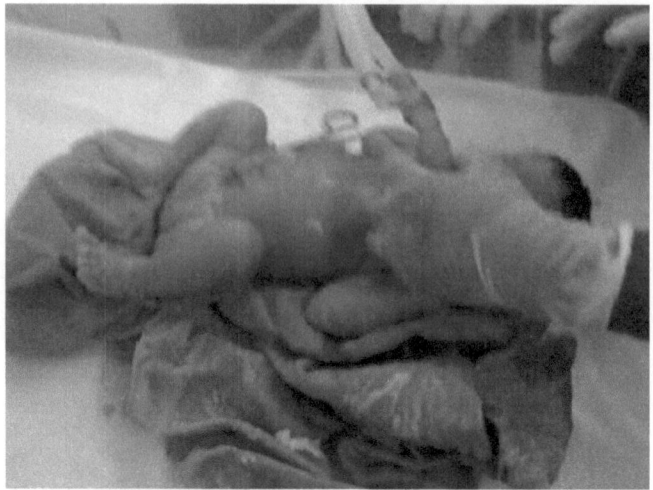

Management of the Pregnant Diabetic

This requires the woman, the obstetrician, physician, and dietician. The drug for managing pregnant diabetics is insulin injection.

The Diabetic in Labour

The children's doctor (paediatrician) will be present during delivery. Prolonged labour should be avoided and the baby monitored closely. Delivery has to be well planned. The woman should notify the staff of the labour or maternity ward of her illness. She should go along to the hospital with a glucometer if she has one.

After delivery:

- She is referred back to the physician
- She is counselled on further pregnancies
- Contraception is discussed to determine the type that is suitable and convenient for her.

CHAPTER 5

THE DIABETIC GOING FOR SURGERY

About fifty percent of diabetics will require surgery at some time during their illness for diabetic complications or other conditions not related to diabetes such as acute appendicitis. Some indications for surgery due to diabetic complications are amputation of a diabetic foot; eye problems such as cataract and proliferative retinopathy; conditions that affect the blood vessels leading to peripheral vascular and coronary artery bypass surgery.

In general, diabetics have poor health compared to those without diabetes mellitus. The diabetic is assessed carefully prior to surgery. Surgery is a form of physical trauma and is frequently accompanied by a period of starvation. Surgical removal of an infected tissue such as amputation of a gangrenous limb, incision of an abscess etc results in reduction in insulin requirement and the danger of low blood sugar during the period after the surgery. Diabetics have a reduced ability to fight infections. Surgery in diabetics is associated with longer hospital stay and greater deaths than in non-diabetics. Increasing evidence shows that high blood sugar levels is associated with poorer outcomes in both diabetics and non-diabetics who undergo surgery. Aggressive blood sugar control positively impacts on the outcome of surgery. The comprehensive risk assessment before the surgery is an important step in the management of the diabetic for surgery.

To make the patient safe for surgery, there is team work between the surgeon, anaesthetist and diabetologist. The surgeon may be a gynaecologist in the case of a woman to undergo gynaecological surgery and an obstetrician in the case of a woman to undergo caesarean section for the delivery of her baby. An anaesthetist is a medical doctor trained to administer anaesthetic agents during a surgical procedure. An anaesthetic is an agent that reduces or abolishes sensation affecting either the whole body (general anaesthetic) or a particular area or region (local anaesthetic).

Diabetic complications such as damage to various organs of the body are important determinants of the kind of anaesthesia to be administered. The risk of significant damage to the body organs increases with the duration of diabetes although the quality of blood sugar control is more important.

Factors Affecting the Management of the Diabetic for Surgery

- Nature of surgery that is if it is a minor or major surgery.
- ➢ Major surgery involves extensive reconstruction or alteration of the body parts and poses great risks.
- ➢ Minor surgery involves minimal alteration in body parts and poses minimal risks compared with major surgeries.

- Urgency of surgery that is if it is an elective or emergency surgery.
- ➢ Elective surgery is scheduled at a time convenient for both the diabetic and the surgeon as the condition requiring surgery is not life threatening.
- ➢ An emergency surgery must be done immediately to save life or preserve function of part of the body.

- Type of diabetes mellitus.
- Usual treatment regimen that is insulin, tablets or diet.
- State of the heart, kidneys and other body organs.

- Level of blood sugar control.
- Type of anaesthesia to be administered.
- Presence of other disease conditions.

Aims of Management of the Diabetic Before, During and After Surgery

- To avoid low blood sugar especially during the surgery
- To avoid excessive high blood sugar
- To prevent the breakdown of fats (lipolysis) and proteins (proteolysis)
- To have good wound healing
- To provide glucose delivery to the tissues

Factors adversely affecting the control of diabetes during surgery are:

- Anxiety
- The response of the body to trauma
- Anaesthetic agents
- Duration of starvation that is the period of fasting on the day of surgery
- Disease underlying the need for surgery
- Other drugs taken by the diabetic for other reasons such as steroids
- Diabetes control prior to admission

The Response of the Body of the Diabetic to Surgery

1. Low blood sugar/glucose (hypoglycaemia)

- This may develop before the surgery is carried out due to the residual effect of some diabetic medications.
- It is worsened by the fasting done on the day of the surgery or insufficient glucose administration.

2. High blood sugar/glucose (hyperglycaemia)

- The response of the body to the stress of surgery and anaesthesia causes an increased secretion of some hormones in the body known as stress hormones whose effects result in high levels of sugar in the blood. These stress hormones are catecholamine, glucocorticoid, glucagon, cytokine, cortisol and growth hormone.
- There is increased breakdown of fats, carbohydrates and proteins during surgery.
- Excess blood sugar in the blood can lead to delayed and impaired wound healing.

Preparation for Surgery

The principles of managing diabetes during surgery depends on the initial (baseline) blood sugar level, level of diabetic control, severity of illness and proposed surgical procedure. Better control of the blood sugar in diabetics undergoing major surgery improves recovery after surgery therefore it is important for the diabetic to be in the best possible condition. The evaluation of a diabetic for surgery assesses the adequacy of blood sugarcontrol, identifies the presence of diabetic complications and other diseases which may have an impact on the outcome of the surgery. The assessment before surgery involves performing some laboratory tests and asking some questions concerning:

- presence of other illnesses such as hypertension
- medications taken for both diabetes and other illnesses
- allergies
- family history of any illness
- previous surgeries and exposure to anaesthesia
- presence of any diabetic complications
- social habits concerning alcohol and tobacco intake
- questions related to the disease requiring surgery.

Laboratory Tests

1. Blood tests

- Estimation of the level of haemoglobin in the blood.
- Fasting blood sugar.
- Test to know the level of some substances in the blood. These are potassium ion, sodium ion, creatinine and urea.
- Glycosylated haemoglobin to assess how well the diabetes is controlled.

2. The urine is tested for:

- protein (proteinuria) as an evidence of diabetic damage to the kidneys known as diabetic nephropathy,
- ketones.

3. Tests to assess the state of the heart in older patients above forty years

- Chest X-ray
- Electrocardiogram (ECG) which is a recording of the electrical activity of the heart on a strip of paper that aids in the diagnosis of heart disease. Electrodes are placed on the skin and connected to the recording apparatus.

4. Tests indicated for the disease requiring the need for surgery.

Diabetics to undergo surgery are admitted 24-48 hours or more prior to surgery for proper assessment and preparation to achieve satisfactory control of the blood sugar. Diabetics require sufficient circulating insulin and glucose to ensure an adequate supply of glucose to the cells in the body.

- For minor surgeries, the diabetic medications are stopped on the day of the surgery. Once the surgery is over, the medications are commenced with the next meal.
- In emergency surgery, insulin injection is started depending on the blood sugar level as there is no time for stabilisation. Emergency surgery is hazardous if the diabetes is poorly controlled.
- Diabetics on tablets (oral hypoglycaemic agents) going for major surgeries are converted to insulin injection. In major surgeries, eating and drinking is not expected to resume by the next meal after the surgery.
- Uncontrolled diabetes must be treated and controlled before elective surgery.

- The diabetic is counselled and a written informed consent for the surgery is obtained. Informed consent is a legal requirement and means that the doctor has informed the individual to undergo surgery of the nature, risks and probable outcome. The individual signs an agreement stating that he or she has been informed and accepts the surgery.

When on hospital admission, the anaesthetist visits the diabetic prior to surgery:

- To establish rapport
- To allay anxiety and fear
- To assess fitness for anaesthesia
- To prescribe certain drugs administered before anaesthesia known as premedication
- To discuss the choice of anaesthesia to be administered
- To correct any misconceptions about anaesthesia.

In elective surgery, normal diabetic medications are taken on the night before the day of the surgery except certain tablets known as long acting oral hypoglycaemic agents that are stopped days before surgery.

Choice of Anaesthesia

- There is no specific guidelines but as dictated by the surgery to be performed.
- The diabetic may either be awake or made to sleep during surgery.
- A regional anaesthetic technique in which the diabetic is awake during surgery is preferred to minimise the response of the body to surgery and anaesthesia, to allow the diabetic communicate

with the doctor in case of symptoms of low blood sugar and helps avoid other anaesthetic problems.

On the Day of Surgery

One of the most important goals in the management of a diabetic for surgery is to minimise the period of starvation, to provide early resumption of normal diet and diabetic medications therefore the diabetic is placed first on the operation list. Breakfast is not taken and a drip containing glucose, insulin and potassium is set on the morning of the surgery.

Artificial devices such as dentures, contact lenses, artificial limbs and big hair piece attachments especially if situated at the back of the head are removed before going to the operating room. Cosmetics are removed from the lips, eyelids and nails because they can mask cyanosis which is the bluish discolouration of the skin and some moist parts of the body such as the tongue due to inadequate amount of oxygen in the blood. The blood sugar is monitored by the doctor during surgery.

Care after Surgery

The care of the diabetic after surgery is aimed at the treatment of pain, maintaining normal blood sugar level, ensuring that there is no bleeding, prevention and early detection of any complication. As soon as eating and drinking resumes, the usual diabetic medications should be commenced. The most important aspect considered in surgery and anaesthesia is the control of the diabetes.

Factors that influence blood glucose sugar after surgery

- Nutritional intake
- Diabetic medications
- Level of activity
- Stress hormones
- Infection
- Pain management
- Psychological state

After surgery, infection at the operation wound site are increased in diabetics especially if the diabetes is poorly controlled. Correct management of the diabetic during surgery reduces the length of hospital admission as well as better wound healing. The diabetic or carer should have resumed control of the diabetes prior to discharge.

CHAPTER 6

THE DIABETIC CHILD

Diabetes is the commonest endocrine disorder seen in children. Diabetes is rare in early childhood although it can still occur. The onset may occur at any age. It affects children of all races worldwide.

Causes of Diabetes Mellitus in Children

The exact cause of diabetes mellitus in children is not known. However, it is due to lack of insulin in the body or inactive insulin being produced in the body.

Management of the Diabetic Child

It is a great shock for parents to be told that their child is diabetic especially if the parents are not diabetic. The management of the diabetic child is multidisciplinary, involving the child, parents, doctor (paediatrician), health educator, dietician, teacher, and other members of the family. A paediatrician is a doctor who deals with children and their illnesses. It is a team work. The condition is explained to the parents. They should keep regular visit on clinic days to allow the health educator to counsel them. The child is actively involved in the management depending on the age. Much parental participation is required because the day-to-day management of their child is in their hands. The child may develop emotional problems when told about the disease. This can manifest as sleeping problems, loss of interest in friends and activities such as sports and school. The child should have a regular feeding pattern.

Medical Treatment

- The child can be managed on diet only. Pure sugars are avoided.
- Insulin is administered. The doctor makes the decision. The child may be admitted into hospital to bring down the high blood sugar level. The parents and child are taught how to inject insulin.
- The parents should note that strenuous physical activity will be dangerous for the child.
- Home monitoring is essential. They should try to have regular supply of needles, syringes, strips, and lancets. It is better to have a personal glucometer for home monitoring of the blood sugar. If they do not have a personal glucometer, the child should have regular blood sugar check in the hospital.
- Psychological support is given to the child and parents.
- Diabetics are susceptible to infections therefore any diabetic child with fever should be seen by a doctor. Self-medication and purchase of drugs over the counter should be avoided. Injection of insulin should not be discontinued when the child is sick. Parents must know that persistent vomiting may require hospital admission.

Parental Support

- The child is encouraged to participate fully in all school activities.
- They should know the symptoms, complications and treatment of diabetes.
- They should know the symptoms and treatment of low blood sugar (hypoglycaemia).
- The school authorities and teacher should be informed on the symptoms and treatment of low blood sugar (hypoglycaemia). If

possible, the child should wear a badge indicating that he or she is diabetic.

- The parents should explain the condition of the diabetic child to the other children in the family. They should all be involved because some children might feel bad because of the extra money spent on the diabetic child's diet and treatment. No special care or interest should develop towards the diabetic child to avoid hatred from other children. All the children in the family should be given equal care and attention.

CHAPTER 7

CONCLUSION

Eating too much sugar is not the cause of diabetes mellitus. Exercising, eating the right food and not being overweight are important. Worldwide, the number of people coming down with diabetes is increasing. Diabetes represents a considerable economic and social burden for the diabetic.

Diabetes mellitus is a chronic disease necessitating lifelong treatment, usually with drugs. This creates a lifelong financial burden on the family especially in low socio-economic communities where the majority of the population still live in poverty. This affects the well being of the entire family, hence the need for early detection, prompt and adequate management of the disease and avoidance of its complications. Diabetics can have a reasonably normal life style. Insulin is the key hormone involved in the storage and controlled release within the body of the energy available from food.

Early diagnosis, correct treatment, and effective follow up are essential to prevent complications and ensure well being. Effective diabetic care is achieved by teamwork. The main aim of treatment is to achieve near normal blood sugar level. The chief principle of diabetic management is to maintain normal blood sugar levels and prevent complications. Diabetes is managed with tablets or administration of insulin injection. Tablets used for the management of diabetes are known as oral hypoglycaemic agents. The pregnant diabetic requires close monitoring. Tight control of the blood sugar in a diabetic going for surgery reduces the rate of infection of the wound and other complications. During ill health in which the diabetic cannot eat or drink for any reason, insulin administration should be continued while monitoring the blood sugar to avoid it being low. Above all, do not stop the drugs without talking to the doctor first.

Minor foot injuries in diabetics can lead to dangerous infections. Many amputations due to diabetic foot could be delayed or prevented by more effective diabetic education and medical supervision. Many diabetic foot problems are avoidable, so diabetics need to learn the principles of foot care and should be advised concerning appropriate foot wear and the risks of smoking. Once tissue damage has occurred in the form of ulceration or gangrene, the aim is to preserve the remaining good tissue. The two main threats are infections and inadequate flow of blood to the foot. Smooth control of diabetes minimises the risk of infection and balances the response of the body to anaesthesia and surgery.

Reduced and loss of consciousness (coma) that requires immediate medical attention develops in severe and inadequately treated diabetes mellitus. The goal of the management of the diabetic going for surgery is to keep the blood sugar as normal as possible. Low blood sugar is potentially damaging at any time and more likely during the surgery because there is increased consumption of glucose by the body in response to surgery. Diabetics are placed first on the operating list to shorten the period of fasting before surgery.

Diabetes is not a death warrant. It is an incurable disease, which can be successfully controlled. There are diabetic associations all over the world where diabetics meet and encourage themselves. Many diabetics have lived healthy lives. Some have undergone surgeries with good outcome. The physical, social, and emotional impact of diabetes and the demands of intensive treatment can create problems for people with diabetes and their families. Join a support group and attend public lectures on diabetes. This will help diabetics to learn about the disease and be encouraged by other diabetics on how they have managed the disease, to know that control is possible and a normal life can be attained. Periodic screening of the populace is important.

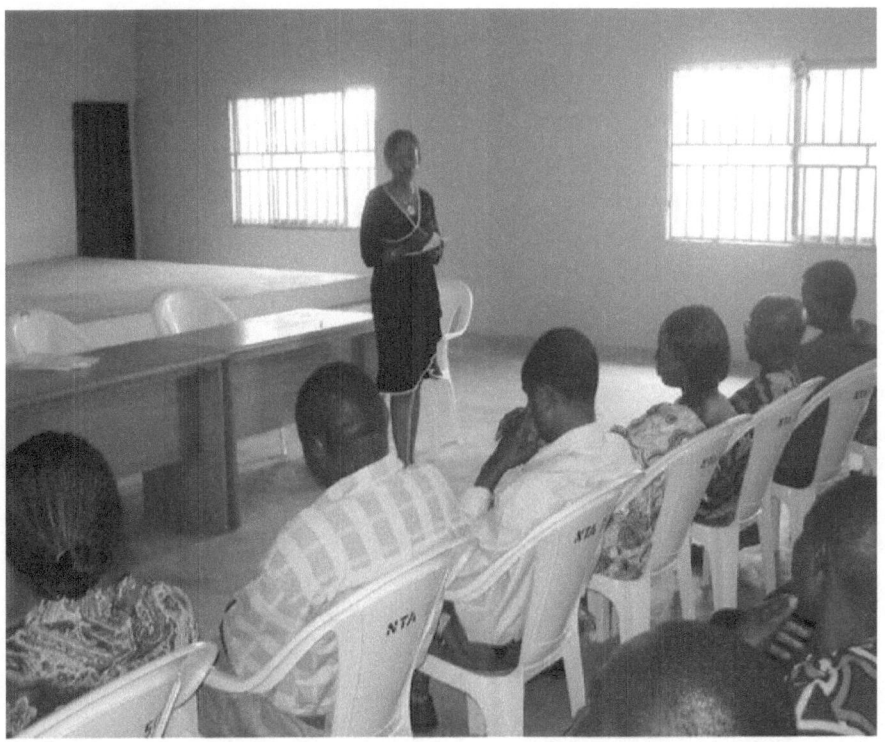

Lecture on diabetes mellitus being given to workers of a media house

REFERENCES

Abioye-Kuteyi EA, Bello IS, Ezeoma IJ, Kolawole BA, Oyegbade OO. Screening for Diabetes Mellitus in a Nigerian Family Practice. South African Family Practice. 2007. 49(8): 15.

Abourawi FI. Diabetic Mellitus and Pregnancy. Libyan Journal of Medicine. 2006. 1(1): 28-41.

Adediran OS, Edo AE. Carbohydrate in Diabetic Diet in Nigeria: is it Evidence Based? The Nigerian Journal of General Practice. 2006. 7(9): 19-23.

Aila Rissanen, Allain Goley, James Gavin. Obesity and Type 2 Diabetes. Synergy Medical Education. 1998.

Akinkugbe OO, Falase AO. A Compendium of Clinical Medicine. Spectrum Books Limited. Ibadan. 2000.

Akinkugbe Ajibayo. A Textbook of Obstetrics and Gynaecology. Evans Brothers Nigeria Publishers Ltd, Ibadan: 1996.

Archampong EQ, Badoe EA, Da Rocha-Afoda JT. Principles and Practice of Surgery. Third Edition. Ghana Publishing Co-Operation, Accra: 2000.

Anochie IC, Eke FU, Opara PI. Childhood Diabetes Mellitus in Port Harcourt: any change in prevalence. Port Harcourt Medical Journal. 2008. 2(2): 126-129.

Bennett Ruth V, Brown Linda K. Myles Textbook for Midwives. Thirteenth Edition. London. Churchill Livingstone. 1999.

Bradley John, Rubenstein David Wayne. Lecture Notes on Clinical Medicine. Sixth Edition. London. Blackwell Publishing. 2003.

Brian McGowan. Churchill Pocket Book of Obstetrics and Gynaecology. Second Edition. London. Churchill Livingstone: 2000.

Carbohydrate. Unilever Educational Booklet Advance Series. 2004.

Clinical Evidence. BMJ Publishing Group. London. 2001. Issue 6.

Chamberlain VPG(ED). Obstetrics by Ten Teachers. Sixteenth edition. London. Bath Press Avon. 1995.

Diabetes: A Guide for South Asian People. British Diabetic Association. 1997.

Diabetic Medicine. 1998. 15 (Suppl 4): S28-S36.

Dunning Trisha. Care of People with Diabetes. Second Edition. London. Blackwell Publishing. 2007.

Elgzyri T. Basic Management of Diabetes Mellitus: Practical Guideline. Libyan Journal of Medicine. 2006. 1(2): 176-184.

Frank WL Ling, Patrick Duff. Pocket Guide for Obstetrics and Gynaecology. London. McGraw-Hill Medical Publishing Division. 2002

Instant Medical Adviser. Career Publishing Inc. New Jersey. 1981.

Malcolm Levene I. Jolly's Diseases of Children. Sixth Edition. India. Blackwell Scientific Publication. 1990.

Michael Clark, Praveen Kumar. Clinical Medicine. Fourth Edition. WB Saunders. 2001.

Miller WFA, Hanretty KP. Obstetrics Illustrated. Fifth Edition. Churchill Livingstone. London. 1997.

Oxford Concise Medical Dictionary. Sixth Edition. Oxford University Press. Oxford. 2003.

Parry EHO(ED). Principles of Medicine in Africa. Second Edition. London. Oxford University Press. 1984.

Savona-Ventura C. Guidelines for the Management of Gestational Diabetes Mellitus. Journal of the Malta College of Family Doctors. 2000.18: 9-12.

Stewart Truswell. ABC of Nutrition. Fourth Edition. London. BMJ Books. 2003.

Tarek Hassan. A guide to Medical Endocrinology. London. Macmillan. 1985.

Velavan J. Surgery and Anaesthesia in Diabetes. In. Shah V, Raji B (Eds). Distance Fellowship in Diabetes Management, a Self-Learning Module for Practitioners. Volume 4. 2010: 57-83.

Watkins Peter J. ABC of Diabetes. Fifth Edition. London, BMJ Books. 2005.

Walsh TS, Pollock AJ. Preoperative Assessment and Preparation. In. Garden OJ, Bradbury AW, Forsythe J (Eds). Principles and Practice of Surgery. Fourth Edition. Elsevier Churchill Livingstone. Philadelphia. 2002. 106-123.

www.changingdiabetes.co.uk

www.diabetes.org.uk